a dive through cancer

by melannie bachman

this book is dedicated
to all beings
impacted by cancer

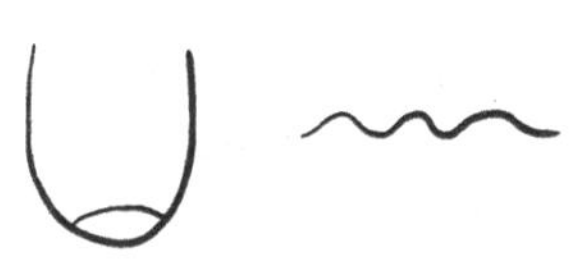

this journey is our journey

Unknowingly, I have been in training to dance
with cancer this entire lifetime. I have come
to accept that one of my gifts is navigating the
underworld. The majority of my life has been
in this high pressure, "uncomfortable"
darkness. Not to mention the ancestral
darkness that lingers in my being. Such
experiences have gifted me the capacity to
navigate life's darkest depths. Instead of
using these experiences as crutches, I use
them as power for connection and love.

Going through this cancer journey has been
deeply profound for me. As a yogi, I have felt
every single piece of it, not only physically,
but emotionally, energetically, ethereally,
ancestrally, collectively and beyond
marinated in every. single. second. Seeing not
only through the eyes, but also the heart in
radical presence.

Having experienced an aggressive breast
cancer diagnosis and treatments, I can
confirm that it is an extremely isolating and
personal journey. Sharing words and
experiences is crucial to bring us back
together through an experience that is so
fractionating. My intention is to inspire
connection, love, hope and healing. To bridge
hearts through the spirit portrayed in these
musings. The pieces are crafted to hone in on
the emotions of my personal journey through
cancer. Less words and more feels. That way,
those going through treatment, are able to
read it. Touching more hearts.

Please acknowledge that everyone's healing
journeys are different, and I share with you

through my lens and heart. I trust in the power of words and more importantly the energy behind them, which I have channeled. Some pieces came through as stories, others as messages, some were abstract. The different voices and styles within this collection of musings has a purpose to connect the variety of community and hopefully at least one of these pieces will touch your heart and bring you to the depths.

May these words root you back to yourself, may they give you a glimpse into the cancer journey, may they help shine light onto what your loved one(s) might be experiencing, and may they bring peace to your journey with the darkness as well as the light. Cancer and treatments is nothing short of the most intense inward journey of your life, if you allow it to be.

In truth, love, depth and light,
Melannie

SHOCK TO THE HEART

welcome to the journey dear one

finding you

valleyed fingertips
sensually caressed my breasts
flirting with eros' boundaries
and what was always known
my soul felt as if it were becoming vapor
as kundalini energy moved up the spine
to the heart
and there you were

a small shock
went through my nervous system
as your shape was examined
hard
small
round
smooth
heart rate increased
my soul jolted down from eros
back to earth
pleasure transmuted to radical presence

i kept you a secret for a few days
to get to know you
feel you
observe you
until i was ready to actualize you

stripped down in the mirror
in-between touching you
and attempting to diagnose you

it is probably nothing serious
then why does it feel that way

my body already knew
it was calling me to find you
the waters just needed to be
still enough
to listen

barrage of testing

fragile skin transmutes
from protecting
to allowing
eventually
the soul becomes numb
to the invasions

out of the mind
and into the body
one needle at a time
never quite knowing the whole picture
rather finding peace in the unknowing
stillness in the swirling
breath becomes life's anchor
with a sublime tranquility in knowing
whatever is
already is

information agitates the mind
as feelings of panic swell
one answer
brings many more questions

can you let it be
can you embody true rooted presence
will you learn to let it go
or choose to struggle
grasping for the unattainable

this life is no different than others
simply new exercises in finding peace
with knowing death
more intimately
than ever explored
herein begin your lessons
with embodied presence

welcome to the journey dear one

peace with departure

if you had a medical diagnosis
that told you death was inevitable
if intervention was not had
would you do it
would you poison your body
for the pain of survival
or would you let it take you peacefully

killing cancer
does not take the pain away from living
it brings you closer to it
so close you can literally taste it

so what to do
who to trust
the journey inward
is only for the courageous
the mystery of life
awaits within
and will take you
beyond
the beyond

deafening diagnosis

unrecognized patterns of numbers
flashed on the screen
it was the long awaited phone call
scrambling to find a quiet place
i answered the call flushed with heat
and quivered hands
through the soundscape
were three words
delivered with such grace

so it's cancer

time froze in deafening silence
the few seconds it took to breathe
felt like an eternity
life was in slow-motion

first to arrive was relief
the peace of knowing
then came fear
sparked from two rooted feet
like a gasoline drenched log meeting a flame
it moved up through the entire body
anxiety quickly suffocated my lungs
and scattered my mind
feeling as if my body were made of glass
shattering
from the increased internal heat and pressure
grief came next
just to produce a single tear
with that liquid release
my body yielded to peace
arriving like moonlit beams
through dark clouds
bathing my soul

the pen and paper dropped from my grip
the doctor's voice hopeful
as she acknowledged
what it may be like to taste such a diagnosis
i'll see you tomorrow
bring your questions
the phone call ended

i was now alone in the room
with the answer
in sublime presence

SLOW IT DOWN TO SET IT FREE

open the heart
journey inward

moving through diagnosis

the body knows how to process
what the mind cannot make sense of

intermittent swirling of nonsensical thoughts
coupled with
the body's innate ancestral knowledge
produces a beautiful dance
between the physical and nonphysical
it is the body that leads us to healing
that brings us to a peaceful seat
alchemizes our emotions
wraps our bleeding hearts
absorbs our tears

following the cancer diagnosis
my body took me for a walk in the darkness
music bathed my soul
as i intuitively moved to the juicy vibrations
making peace with contrasting emotions
shifting trauma through and out of the body
making space to receive healing
that was ready to arrive
we sang
we cried
we healed
together dancing
mind with body

waking the next morning
feeling half alive
with swollen eyes
and a sore heart
i arrived to the doctor's office
placed in a room with a large circle table
encouraged to record the conversation
as the doctor somehow knew
that the mind gives way to the body
after receiving such a diagnosis
with notepads in hand
my partner and i arrived
to our seats at the table
two binders were placed in front of us

worn as if they were used far too often
but now it was our turn
treatment plans were delivered in flow charts
laminated pages holding more than just ink

this diagnosis cannot belong to me
i felt disbelief
as if they were delivering this news
to the wrong person
there were only two options
no more
no less
leaving me in a state of awe
death was implied
but never spoken of
although it quietly sat on my shoulders
making its presence felt in the room for all

how can people afford this
the cost of treatment so astronomically high
it was not even discussed at the appointment
the mind so full of information
with no way to process it beyond the breath
here is where i began to learn
to take each moment
one step at a time
one day
one hour
one minute
one second
one breath

here are your selected doctors
your oncologist will see you next
you're so young for cancer
let's run your genetic panel today

two shaking cold hands held tightly
to a stack of pamphlets and information
for this new designation of
cancer patient
wobbly legs carried my body to get the first
of countless
blood draws

as the body began to move
the stuck emotions felt their opportunity
to also move

i was called back into a dark room
with no windows
my body welcomed by a cold black seat
smelling of rubbing alcohol
the nurse prepped my arm

i have cancer
i said it out loud
tasting how it felt
coming off my tongue and out my mouth
it felt like a shock to the system
as truth integrated in the body
emotions erupted like a dam release
from mind to body
the phlebotomist met my emotions
without will
she was physically thrown back
the needle ripped out of my arm
and cut my skin as blood decorated the seat
my clothes
and the room
just as my emotions had
both of us aware of the energetic sonic boom
that just knocked us both
out of this physical realm

she apologetically prepped again
flustered
showering me with prayer
tears welling in her eyes
as she wished me love
knowing we may never meet again
i left the room
covered in dark sticky reds

can I find home here
underwater in this deep dark cave
of the messy unknown
moving through diagnosis
transmuting energy

from mind to matter
to the depths of being
one with diagnosis

slow drip

it can be that simple
but will you allow it to be
cancer slows us down
with such beauty
one is able to feel more
see more
be more
there is magic in the pace
and if allowed
it will teach us
how to relax
simplify
to see love as it truly is
the simplicity of being with love
in stillness

will you allow it to open your heart
to the abundance
that is overflowing
washing over the body's myriad of cells
allowing us to see the connection
between all living things

such a parallel symbol of peace is the forest
a beautiful tapestry of tempo
abundant life in the stillness
the forest is elegant
simple
love
peace
accepting
gracious
nurturing
and she is
because of her speed

to slow down enough
to feel the raindrop's journey
from the collected waters above
down the protective bark
to the depths below
rooted and entwined

anchored
connected
strong
here is where you find
what you have been searching for

it takes more than open eyes
to feel
to be
to embody
the essence of peace
on slow drip

lessons in letting go

experiencing a life threatening diagnosis
illuminates our attachment to life

attachment
enlightens
detachment

release is an embodied practice
it cannot be done solely through the mind
letting go is layered
mind within
body within
soul

fear of release
paralyzes
clinging to advice
immobilizes

close down the eyes
be still
open the heart
journey inward
move
breathe
express attachments
allowing them a gracious exit
and eventually
release will become familiar
like an old friend

allow it to be effortless
journey
through
where
magic
abounds
again and again

LIFT ME UP

will you walk with me

my tribe

people continually surprise me
with grand love
appearing in ways never imagined
providing lessons in pure abundance
constantly blown away by
true kindness
unparalleled generosity

it was community
that wrapped me in light
embraced me
accompanied me
by working together
in divine play
every person accepting their role
and each role so very different
no one person could orchestrate
such an amalgamation of gifts
for a common purpose

it is pure beauty
divine flow
this tribe
is the nature
of unbounded love

your story is our story

we met in a hallway
waiting for our turns
with the overbooked oncologists
our souls connected
with a lock of the eyes
innate knowing
i was placed to hear your story

father
son
african american
alone
living with incurable blood cancer
you poured your heart into mine

a story of hopelessness
heartbreak
strength
grieving the death of your mother
who passed of breast cancer
then receiving a cancer diagnosis yourself
days later
losing your job due to a pandemic
your home due to someone else's greed
you were left alone
but full of faith
slowly allowing the pieces
to come back together
stronger than before
the resilience
you broke
and rebuilt stronger
like kintsugi

you stand tall sharing with me
hope gleams from your eyes
overpowering the apparent pain
aspiration for another day
for more time
for this precious gift of life

your story emulated through the halls
to the ethers
like a fine golden mist
finally set free

through feeling your story
my heart ached
i lost my breath
tears welled in my naked eyelids
i could taste your despair
while also feeling your courage

your story of hope
strengthened me
it showed me that i needed some
your faith still radiates through me
as a beautiful reminder
that your story
is our story

ode to my lover

will you walk with me
support my side body so i will not fall
share with me what happens
when the world does not stop turning
distract me from the pain
show me what you see from your lens
will you simply be
allow me to observe you
to witness life's fluid nature
while i embody
a reflection pond of still waters

like a chameleon
i move in slow motion
attentive to earth's most delicious moments
i can feel your heartbeat
see the trepidation in your eyes
observe your soul through its vessel

will you remind me what it is like to laugh
remind me why i am still alive
to fill me with faith
for just another moment
until my next slumber
when i journey further inward to new realms
the light you cast back
is a mirror
grateful for the reflection
one i can feel
not just see
absorb
but not fully understand
it reminds me
i am held
i am seen
i am alive
this reflection
through
your being

DEATH REQUIRED FOR LIFE

because of you
i am free

the chair

there you stood
tan and grand
sterile with a tag to claim so
made for holding frail bodies
designed to embrace us through the experience

you will be in chair #8 today
a magical number for me
the number of infinity
i felt the divine essence in your embrace
as i took my seat
i fell backwards
yielding into you
surprised at how you caught me
with your cold firm pleather gummed casing

would you like a blanket
the nurse asks
i nod in approval
unsure of whether this is a standard offering
but later i learn it is to assist the chair
in softening its embrace
and to warm the chilled bodies it holds

a footrest
a table
you had it all
as i look around
no one else smiled in your muted embrace
the others looked depleted
hopeless
pale
lonely
defeated
in your large sterile hug
you held us safe
asking nothing in return
a place to find comfort
in the uncomfortable

brown bag

hours are spent waiting to hear
if i passed pre-health screenings
to receive brown bag
a small internal celebration arrives
as the nurse declares me clear
to receive treatment
cold alcohol bathes my chest port site
smelling fierce as my senses are heightened
with the nerves of anticipation
a sharp burning stab of lidocaine arrives
taking a deep breath in
i exhale pain out
the port is then accessed
feeling like a ribcage invasion
the pressure so strong
as if the goal is to force the air out of my lungs
with a thick needle
a quick flushing of the port device
gives sensations in a spot never felt before
somewhere between the skin
heart
lungs
and tastes of strong concentrated plastic
arriving from the bottom of my throat
into my mouth

the body must be prepped to receive chemo
each step carries its own importance
after my port is connected to the pumps
the hydration bag is hung and delivered
then oral medications are administered
assuring less adverse effects to brown bag
different prep for different chemo
my patience is tested
waiting for brown bag
barely breathing
mostly observing
fully feeling
while also numb
holding unease high in my chest
the nurses stir quickly
as the awaited brown bags are delivered

to each patient
it is a loud circus of checkmarks
so much fuss
to make sure the correct bag
is delivered to the proper patient
my skin begins to tighten as i await my turn
the nurse arrives again and this time gowns
in full protective equipment
to ensure none of the brown bag
touches her skin
it is my turn
the medicine comes double bagged
with loud safety warnings on every bag
brown covers protect the chemo medicine
as it is powerful yet sensitive to light
two nurses check every detail
verbally declaring out loud
the medication and dosage
with the patient name
again making sure this brown bag is yours
and yours alone

they finally hang my brown bag
i label it with a pink post-it note
magic juice
to assure my being this is going to heal me
some call it poison
but i choose to believe it is medicine
flow rate is set
and the nurses leave

now alone with my thoughts
emotions
fears
anxiety
sadness
confusion
loneliness
multiple hours waiting
feels like days alone in the desert
breathing in patience and breathing out fear
each second feels like a lifetime
constantly scanning my body for symptoms
for reactions to the brown bag

listening to others' reactions
to their brown bags

will that happen to me

but then i put two tiny plastic buds in my ears
crank up the music
summoning the divine for strength
for my body to accept the medicine
for the healthy cells to survive
for the cancer cells to leave
in the most intense wait and see game
of my life
completely out of control
feeling anxiety swirling in my cells
while holding strength
fiercely living in duality

that color of brown
is forever ingrained in my memory
when i see it in the world
i think of brown bag
all the people it has helped
all the people it has killed
all the research that went into creating it

for me
brown bag held new beginnings
of life beyond
a two year expiration date

the first dose

waiting
lying in bed
too sick to stand
peering out the window
feeling in a prison of one's own body
knowing that this first dose
is inside the cells
already administered
with no turning back
only moving forward
it is a fear and a peace
a lack of control
with only layers of acceptance
in the anticipation
of sickness

was it too much they gave me
was it just enough to stop the cancer
how do i know
what do i expect

alone
laying with thoughts
consumes
as each passing moment
weakens the body further
the sun becomes blinding
as if its life giving rays
could cause demise
from just existing near their radiance
it is the feeling of every bodily cell
dying

how can it get worse
i am so afraid of a slow death like this

there is still faith in the form of hope
hope that this miraculous body
will survive the storm
the sacred vessel
holding the soul safe

sorrow arrives
washing over the body as sadness
the internal knowing that this
is poisoning of the body
electively

the cancer wants to replicate
how is there harm
in something that seems so innocent
my body is just good at growing cells

the eyes finally close on inhale
yielding to the lack of control
on exhale
the ultimate release occurs
from the utmost hidden places
never felt before within the body
rest brings healing
as feelings pause
dream state is welcomed

excitement arrives when the pain
stops accelerating
a small smile cracks
from the sides of the mouth
as ease swells

maybe this was the worst of it

rising feels like a hard stumble
the endurance of sickness
is unrivaled
only those who have journeyed through
can understand
what it is to be caught in the mind
body
emotion
communing with poison
making friends with darkness
hoping for life
and most times
praying for death

dancing with the red devil

i now understand
the nickname *red devil*
staring at me through that large syringe
those artificial red kool aid hues
resemble poison
during your journey
straight into my heart

are you red to alert others of your toxicity
of your potency to cancer cells
are you red to remind nurses to deliver slowly
at just the perfect rate
are you red because you attack the heart
as some hearts arrest upon your arrival

these thoughts spew through my mind
every time i see you
once the short plastic hose is connected
to the opening in my aorta
we begin

unable to watch you enter my body
i look away
full of complete terror
unable to breathe
tears well and stream down my cheeks
receiving you is pure trauma
no matter how much i have prepared my soul
and attempted to convince myself
that you are medicine
you frighten me
my heart races as the countdown continues
i feel you enter my arteries
as you burn on occasion
like fire slicing through my vasculature
i gaze out the window
crank the tunes louder in my ears
but nothing can distract me
the entire 15 minutes you enter my blood
a tickle of tears stream down my cheeks
my whole body trembles
i literally drown in my own fear

connected to you with no turning back
knowing what you will take from me

i feel the tug of the syringe disconnecting
that is my cue that i can return my gaze
the nurse removes her protective coverings
i am finally able to take a deep breath
as if I took the deepest dive of my life
that sweet deep relief
of fresh oxygen
bathes over me
washing me clean of you

my swollen salty eyes
remind me of your *power*
i continue to expel you
through my neon colored urine
for days to come
i am toxic waste
and every release of you from my body
tears
sweat
spit
are all poisonous to others
and demand sterilization to protect loved ones
from your touch
red devil

my skin turns yellow
after our infusion together
but at least the trauma of receiving you is over
now courage must rise
with both internal and external vibrations
i must stay strong
it is the only way
to survive the *red devil* for the weeks ahead

the challenge in receiving you
builds a warrior
i transform my deepest of fears
to the strongest roots of courage
it is how i dance with you *red devil*

there is a lifetime limit
of how many encounters we can share
and for us
we had our final dance

thank you
for all the lessons
learning how to separate
from the trauma
emotions
pain
in order to stay unattached
and survive
learning to live
through poison

thank you
for dismantling my angst
and my tumor
maybe those red tones
resemble more than your nickname
rather blood
life force
root chakra
i survived you
in exchange
for a longer life
bathed in the beauty of red

a sea of medications

my world is surrounded
with a sea of medications
fabricated in laboratories
some designed to alleviate the others
while others work to intensify
each with a purpose

i unscrew the lids
guzzle them down
like it means nothing
completely detached
from the enormity of it all
feeling captivated by their spells
numb to their influence over my body
numerous pages in a journal
document my symptoms
more artificial substances than natural
now live in my body
i was resistant to medications at the start
but doubled over in pain
i eventually grasped for their crutch
for just a taste of relief
even for a second
this is the time to
fight medicine
with medicine

the collection of pharmaceuticals grow
as my symptoms intensify
lying on the bathroom floor
fetal position
paralyzed by pain
so detached from a feeling of natural
all i feel is malaise
void from the inside out
my soul has disconnected from my body
to help lessen the amount of pain that is felt
although i feel numbed out
unaware that you left me

emotions are clouded
nothing matters
this void weaves with intense feelings
fused together
medications with body
waiting for a clear day ahead
in an existence
free from this
internal prison
guarded by the artificial sea

fertility fears

sitting here is surreal
a place of differing paths
joined in the fertility journey
a young woman with her mother
with faces of fear
older couples with hope
and me
confused
numb

i do not belong here

knowing death is about to consume me
this is the logical next step
protecting fertility
brought into an office
filled with photos of smiling families
children everywhere

what am i doing here

papers handed over for review
statistic after statistic
i was now a number
no longer a person
with a greater chance of death than life
overwhelmed by the process
doubting its alignment

this is not how humans naturally conceive
are we forcing life

feelings drop away
as the body leads
too much to absorb
a receptionist declares
the financial commitment due
within a few days
greater than the cost of a luxury vehicle
with little to no guarantee it will work

are you kidding me
this is the only system

i am filled with rage
heartbreak
confusion
and brought back to stillness
to listen
trust
be
in the unknown
with the wounds
of my womb
the seat of power
love
life
and soon to be
death

death

like an eerie mist
death travels through the body
bringing awareness
to the unknown facets
it flows as if on a mission
elegant
the movement is unrivaled blinded beauty
to be known intimately
unapologetically
fiercely intense
yet soft

death has an unforgettable taste
it rises up from the deep internal seat
and is met at the back throat
a taste of rot
textured of slime and dehydration
feeling strong for days
the tongue whitens as cells perish
food unable to mask the taste

death encroaches through the nostrils
into the sinus cavities
the nares
where it can be smelled
flowing out of the skin's pores
as it exits from the body
eliciting feelings of decomposing
from the inside out

can anyone else smell this

it then ventures to the eyes
where pressure and pain are overwhelming
relief only when the eyelids shut
as the eyes crave darkness
after meeting death
each organ's lining deeply aches
the throat
heart
lungs
diaphragm

stomach
spleen
kidneys
liver
intestines
bones
joints
blood
fascia
womb space
rest is the only thing welcomed
as spirit detaches from the body
during the days of encroaching death

the doctors' prescription is to move
to walk through the pain

one foot in front of the other
the body maneuvers
through bone crushing pain
into the deep unknown
focusing on steps
barely breathing
eyes half closed
the body mourning itself
cells attempting to escape the fog of death
the body working in extreme conditions
dying to survive
surviving to die
that is the dance of cancer

bellowing at times for death
it is impossible to avoid a relationship with it
approaching the limits
feels painful yet blanketed in peace
a universal space
where time is of no existence
and suffering becomes grace

the vapor of essence
in this place of nothingness
the comfort of the darkness
where the light shines brightest
and just before fully releasing here

life returns yet again
and the darkness gently lifts
as if evaporating
into the colorless ethers of light
the pain subsides
as the soul returns to the body
not yet fully rooted
but rather a subtle reuniting
feeling physically stronger
no longer tasting death
but very much remembering it

death begins to feel so familiar
as if coming home
to a deeper part of self
to a place where time stands still
peace abounds
and fear no longer exists

death is so pungent
but also so sweet
those who have traveled here
know this place well
and our cells forever remember it

dear death
thank you for teaching me
how to endure
thank you for the reminder
of the beauty of you
and in life
of the deeply rooted
unparalleled strength
within us all
because of you
i am free

LONELINESS TOGETHER

without brings you within

waiting room

most days the floor welcomed me
as an abundance of patients
occupied every waiting room chair

looking around the room
i saw sadness
defeated spirits
severe sickness
bodies closer to death than life
weakness shown in the glazed personas
almost every head bowed in defeat
eyes half open
breath hardly audible
no speaking
so quiet
in community
yet so alone

my body drained from chemotherapy
slouched on the stained carpet
resting against tacky wallpaper
i managed to crack a smile
to the unmet gazes
alone in our togetherness

but then a light appeared
she was an angel
in a pastel sky blue colored dress
floor length and baggy
her bald head wrapped neatly
in a beautiful soft pink floral scarf
cooler in hand and large bag in the other
she was prepped for a long day of infusion
there was something special about her
her soul beamed out to the others in the room

i am celebrating
she declared out loud
it was her final chemotherapy infusion
my heart raced in excitement for her
it already felt as if she was family
as if it were my last treatment too

that will be me one day
i hold onto that hope
that ray of light in a room of darkness
thank you blue dressed angel
for wearing your heart
for smiling under your mask
for your hope
your bravery

your celebration
is our celebration

wrapped in light

like a switch
all attention is on you
and then no more
on then off
where is everyone
questions arise out of fear
then are left unanswered

how does a bird learn to fly
but to be pushed out of the nest
as we too must learn
to journey through a solitary season
by a free fall into the fire
out of it arises
a strengthening of self
character
love
faith
trust
hope
connection
a phoenix
from the ashes
to assure us
that we are all connected

keep breathing dear one
feel the sweetness of each sip
the release of each exhale
breath is a cycle
of receiving
and letting go
nourishing
expelling
bound by love
and timeless
you my dear
are prana wrapped in light
remember
without brings you within

escaping eros

a place where divinity flourishes
with the union of souls
sacred
powerful
an expression of life
love
the juice of life itself
finally found
yet broken down
so quickly

touch feels painful
instead of pleasurable
connection feels unattainable
to self or another
eros goes absent
nowhere to be found
it is as if the heavenly portal
has been bolted shut
frustrated
angry
grieving
pleasure alchemizes into pain

the body has adapted
to killing cancer cells
for survival
not for celebrating life
tears fill bare eyelids
as multiple attempts
to find pleasure in touch
are denied

*where is the beauty
in this sea of pain*

pleasure experiences death
just as the body does
the root chakra ember
does not blaze from expectations
eventually returning
only to be found

in new
unexplored places
from a deeper place within

patience
pleasure is intricately connected to pain
it is a complex network
give it space
to surprise you
upon eros return
a shock
to the heart
deeply rooted
will be felt
and revered
now evermore connected
pain with pleasure
eros in its entirety

energy's power

energy is so powerful
we forget
sometimes
there are no words
no acts of service
no items
no money
no explanations
no complexities
no right or wrong
no good or bad
no labels
no answers
no time
no no

OUT WITH THE OLD IN WITH THE NEW

in losing you
i found me

triumphant tresses

it took some time for death to release you
the anticipation of losing you
stalked my dreams
followed me throughout my days
burning of the scalp
preceded your death

i felt you die
the moment you went limp
after that first dose
it started slow
like a heavy shedding
but then accelerated
within hours
you were falling out by the handfuls
you made it known
it was time
whatever was left on my scalp
was merely waiting
for its turn to drop
an energetic disconnect occurred
which aided in the removal from my body
but did not help with the emotional pain

with every vibrating pass of the trimmers
my body trembled in feelings

was it grief
the fear of being fully seen
or the pain of no control

more like a messy combination of it all
wrapped heavily in peace
tears fiercely fell
in a steady stream
as release took place
i was shedding my skin
like a snake
a rebirth
new sensations overwhelmed my senses
as i traveled to the unknown

there is no hiding here
facing the world with total humility
the falling of an ego
a byproduct of chemotherapy pain
such a humbling freedom of who was
of what had been
of where there was to go
completely bare
from the outside in

that breath sure felt tasty
after your last drop
relief radiated my entire being
it washed over me
like coming clean
this was revival
unattached
the ultimate simplicity
freedom
hope
courage

in losing you
i found me

shedding gratitude

the extravagant layers
wrapped around each one of your strands
you have seen the world with me
from mystical seas deep underwater
to volcanic mountain tops

drenched in salt crystals
all the stories you have witnessed
the adventures you felt
from the heat of indonesian soil
to the thick marshes of old villages

you held a lovers' tug of passion
the oceans' power from waves overhead
sunrises in remote island huts
diving dreads from mask straps
absorbed copious salty tears
and hours of sweat soul grounding on the mat

you were an extension of me
your beauty framed my soul
although it did not define it

my deepest gratitude
dear locks of love

without you

i now face this world
completely naked
amazed at how much
hair covered
in my being
the complete vulnerability
in sickness
and strength
the deepest i have ever been
surrounded in the greatest love
ever witnessed
experiencing the highest highs
and lowest lows
intertwined in
every
single
moment

life feels powerful
sickness feels daunting
love feels expansive
this
this is life on burning coals
this is life poets and artists portray
and now
i can finally see the rawness of beauty
feel its vibration
so emotionally delicious

bald beauty

release was the hardest part
surprisingly
acceptance came easy

softer than silk
touching my bald head
was pure joy
amazed by new sensations
constantly chilled
easily satisfied
slathered bassu oil
gave reflective textures
that sure met gazes
encountering this world hairless
felt extraordinarily familiar

in baldness i felt fierce
the true embodiment of an ego's fall
there was no hiding behind a frame
it was complete freedom
cageless
with rays of childlike enthusiasm
that beamed from my crown

it felt as if i was reborn
walking the earth with new skin
like an infant from the womb
a reminder that underneath it all
was me awaiting
to appreciate
love and accept
the raw
beauty
of truth

ceremonial burn

wrapped in tiny rubber bands
you rested in a sacred box atop the altar
i pulled you out
caressed you over my upper lip
just to see how you felt for the final time
one more deep inhale of your essence
it was intoxicating
i placed you in the ceremonial basket
specially picked for this moment
the fire was roaring
she beckoned for you
the flames burned bright
reminding me of ethereal power

it was time for the ceremonial release
i created a sacred space
the deck illuminated with candles
sprinkled in gold dust
flowers and sentimental items
adorned the space
crystals shimmered in the fire's flicker
music weaved it all together with the ethers

under electrical stars
we created communion
a blessing of body and soul
first i fed the flames
with healing talismans
that assisted me in my cancer journey
candles
cards
photos
the tribal love
i joyfully received it
and released it back to the cosmos

then came the basket of my hair
my most attached piece
you called for it
and i obeyed
with a heart of peace wrapped in affliction
i laid your silky strands serenely

in the basket
and lowered you into the flames

i watched as you met with fire
there was no reaction at first
rather an amalgamation of energies
then came the moment
hair joined with fire
smoke swirled in the union
the flames crackled
changed colors
it was such an honor to witness
as i finally found my breath
in the creation of ash

i released you back to the divine mother
no longer grasping you
fearing your loss
or waiting for death
but in full acceptance
encircled in love
a visible departure
from earth
to pachamama
the bellowing of thunder blanketed the sky
as the offerings moved upward
towards abundance
clouds quickly moved in overhead
sounds of ancestral drums roared overhead
until rain poured from the dark sky
washing the ceremonial space clean
soothing the raging fire
welcoming the rebirth

such a magical experience
to become so integrated
with life and death
receiving
releasing
the pure sweetness of divinity
left with nothing
yet having everything

moon cycle magic

housed in the sacred womb space
two tiny yet mighty organs
hold power to create life
both sacral and root chakras
mingle where the ovaries rest
wearing their cloak of protection
vibrational mantra and sacred talismans
in blessed mala beads and roses
shielded the divine feminine
energetically
spiritually

both ovaries were placed
in medicinal slumber
preventing their ancient cycles
safeguarding them from ravenous chemo
monthly intense stings of injections
kept them asleep
after chemotherapy was complete
their awakening process was safe to begin
the womb struggled
to pulse with her natural rhythm
finding it again after 249 days
in perfect timing
my womb welcomed its sacred bleed
from the intense pull of a supermoon
release was found

shedding of more than the mind could imagine
all that the body needed to discard
housed in red
feelings of relief
tears of unrivaled joy
a reconnection back to earth
to the divine mother
the chance at fertility
the return of kundalini power
simplistic awe
of the magic
and power
of menstruation

body blessing

this body is a gift
a sacred vessel
cherished beyond comprehension
what a privilege to bless this body
such energetic medicine
aligns soul with spirit
producing deeply rooted strength
with wild courage

through cancer
all this body endured
needle sticks
hoses inserted
fluids and tissues removed
organs cut apart
medicines pumped in
radioactive dyes absorbed
countless scans of invisible toxic waves
and never a complaint
sure this body felt pain
but it always prevailed stronger
accepting of change
adapting graciously

we joined to bless this body
in community
but also as an inward journey
with lighted chakra candles on the altar
breath guided energy's direction
in complete trust of the body as a teacher
the body was acknowledged
appreciated
revered

strength propelled us forward
in change together
gracefully
in love and full receivership
of the great esoteric mystery

synthetic breasts

the complexity of emotions
overwhelm my system
i see your silicone circles in my mind's eye
under the skin
holding place of where my breasts once were
touching you is different
lacking feeling
with random electrical shocks of pain

i move you in the pocket
like squeezing a hard water balloon
a loss of connection
between the skin and my heart
you feel different in water
no longer softening in water's embrace
touching you is now cold
with hints of thin warmed skin
tracing the breasts' past existence
is full of lumps
numbness plays where nerves once lived
i trace my fingers over the horizontal scars
where my nipples were
tears well and drop as i am reminded
of what was taken from me
disposed of as medical waste

grief arrives
with awareness
of how attached to the physical body i am
i will never get to feel natural breasts again
or the connection of a baby's latch
yet i breathe in love
and breathe out the attachment
i trace the scars in remembrance
feeling the sadness of losing an organ
the love of your memory
and the complexity
of all that is
in-between

THE UNKNOWN OF REBIRTH AND HEALING

how do you begin again

body image

this new shape i carry
swollen spongy skin
curves fresh and expanding
how gorged these cells have become
with extra fluid from treatments

how come it took changing shapes to see it

i feel shame for under appreciating
the body's strength all these years
i slide one leg into the denim pant
and immediately feel truth
still in denial
i thread the other
unable to even shimmy it to my hips
this body has expanded
she is taking up more space
i sit on the bed
sorrow washing over me
not for outgrowing my jeans
but because i ignored
this body's innate power for so long
sadness as i think of all she has endured
and that it has taken me this long
to truly listen

graciously i pull one leg out at a time
fold the denim on my bed
and stand in front of the full length mirror
tracing these new shapes with my fingertips
appreciating her
this body's strength
resilience
love for me
this sacred vessel
what a gift

hand on womb i cry to her in love
asking what this new shape needs
she replies quickly

soft and flexible

i answer in action
off to the store
to find the most comfortable leggings
designed to hold
and hug her new expansive shapes
i am led to the soft mottled pink
first pair
first wear
it is perfect

this body will never look the same
a rebirth brings changes
total transformation
inside and out
this body showcases impermanence
wearing her with breathtaking beauty

*why do we fight so hard
denying what is*

as i change
she changes
may we flow together
in this divine union
body and soul
pure love
in all our shapes

the wild unknown

undomesticated
this realm feels foreign
yet all too familiar
seeded deep within these cells
are the wild codes
yet returning to them
feels like an uncomfortable journey
traveling deep into the self
through the pain
through the lack of control
through the anxiety
through the fear
through the numbness
through the darkness
to reach the electricity
the vibrancy
the technicolor
the raw
the fierce
the exhilaration
the bountiful
omnipresent
pure spacious divinity
a place
few have ventured
into the intoxicating darkness
where light is magic
inhales become cavernous
as rooted exhales anchor
this is
the wild

sweet taste of rebirth

an exponential feeling
of relief
regeneration
electricity
shooting from all cells
back into the world
joy abounds
magnifies
radiates
death is forgotten
as light prevails
wildly luminous

could I just stay here awhile longer

rebirth is addicting
fiercely sweet
exhilarating
and impermanent
accompanied by death
cyclical
everlasting
unending
the elixir
of skeleton woman

depression's hold

latched onto my heart
i feel darkness
leaching through my entire being
it must find joy in suppressing my spark
feeding off my light
the lows feel like an unending drop
with intermittent pauses
that bring awareness to pain
tears release depression's hold for a moment
then it finds a way back in
over and over again
this dis-ease of darkness

can anyone see this pain i am fighting inside

so invisible
yet upfront and driving my life
nothing feels familiar
except for this darkness
like an old friend
i cling to it like a security blanket
it feels of an older version of self
the one who kept me awake at night
to protect me from violence

we grew so close together
delight and affliction
there must be a part of me
that finds pleasure in pain
numb to the world around me
the discomfort feeds my erratic mind
triggers my reactive emotions
all to keep me spiraling in the void

they do not warn you
cancer recovery requires stamina
not only physical
but emotional
others hide away in their silence
suppressed by their own inner darkness
feeling the tenacity of the underworld
as the mind seems to recover quicker

than the physical body
giving depression its fuel
and the darkness
its hold

but then i am reminded of life's beauty
in the innate simplicities
from a slight breeze
in the air displaced by a dragonfly's wings
gentle and swift
i allow the light in through the cracks
and through the softest illumination
the shadow is pierced

i feel you sweet soul
this dance with darkness
it is how we learn fortitude
traveling through the depths
but that is where the light
shines most magical
when you look up
from the depths below

fatigue

some days feel as if
i am an empty shell housing a soul
as if all physical energy needed to operate
has been sucked away
with each morning's sunrise
hope arrives for fuel
then eventually
after hundreds of days in a row
acceptance arrives
for this new normal

the exhaustion is like no other
tiredness finds its way through
muscle
skin
organs
the heart
every cell feels drained of life
it hits differently than depression
like a systemic lack of existence
too weak to think
or move
to feel emotions
or survive
completely invisible to others
the intensity is confusing
beyond nothingness

what is life
i survived cancer for a life like this
was treatment worth it

relief feels fictitious
living in a prison
no one can see
more than a difficult time
it is death on slow drip
softly excruciating
suffocating
with one thing left
to be
depleted

alone
forgotten
with not even
a

.

rediscovering myself

i was led to a magical place
she called to me through the ethers
in lush greens and rusted browns
hugged by forest giants
held safe in their long branches
i bathed in the trees
and felt at home for the first time
since this journey began

i am a reborn wanderer
with presence to guide me
i float where the wind and earth move me
trusting the pulsating power
of interconnection
previous labels to my being have been shed
burned in the flames
unsure of what comes next
guided by a deeply awakened intuition
more connected than ever
yet also aware of disconnect
in this wild unknown territory

how do you begin again

with each step forward
rebirth empowers a choice
a new pace through life
recalibrating to nature's tempo
instead of societal speed
no longer returning to former ways
it is essential to reclaim your power
trust the process
listen with more than your ears
feel with every ignited cell
essence as divine vapor
return to ancient ways
it may feel foreign and new
but it has always
been you

a story of aletheia

pain became such a friend
it took up so much residence
i was accustomed to it
as a part of me
like the clothes i wore daily
until it finally occurred
i could let the affliction go

my body was telling me all along
how come i refused to fully listen
the full body malaise
sharp and dull chronic pains
joint aches
menstrual irregularities
debilitating pelvic pain
depression
swollen body
tired eyes
severe exhaustion
eros disconnect
feeling as if my body was attacking itself
the doctors labeling this
as my *new normal*

like a slow death
from the inside out
my body was rejecting
the silicone implants placed within
from every cellular level
i was drowning in pain
but unable to see it

numbly following the ways of those before
blindly trusting the doctors' advice
who have personally never walked this path
i was stuck moving in no direction
with unknown coordinates
hopeful that with each procedure or surgery
relief would come
yet it never did
complication after complication
i finally had enough

choosing to be finished
with breast reconstruction
was the ultimate relief
i had prioritized my body's health
it felt unchained
empowering to vocalize my truth
to myself
doctors
surgeons
nurses
other survivors
this was the moment
when depth of healing began

chest surgery felt different this time
a deconstruction rather reconstruction
less postoperative sickness
more joy
that first deep breath post surgery
was pure nirvana
i anchored into the feeling of health
ease
lightness
peace
truth
deep into my womb
sealing it into my being

i let the waves of grief resurface
but it was different this time
after the rush passed
healing anchored in
i was no longer spiraling in the feelings
truth was the ultimate grounding

i let my body reveal itself to me
it took six days to feel ready
to look down at the incisions
alone in a sacred space
with only candles
a mirror
and aletheia
i gazed at my body
my truth

through a salty lens of tears
i touched the fresh incisions
the closest my hands have ever been
to my heart
feeling so exposed
but yet so whole
healed
and finally free
ready
to move
forward

at times i feel shame
wondering why
i electively poisoned my own body
not ready to bear
the full anguish of losing a body part
but i needed to walk all the steps
to feel the entire journey
i may have never appreciated my truth
without the experiences in-between
they were all simply the layers
around loving
and losing my breasts

fingertips trace
the hills and valleys of my ribcage
indents of where my breast used to live
my heart beats are now visible to the world
these are scars of a warrior
i survived death
for life
no longer housing an artificial organ
under my skin
i am able to wear my truth
representing all i have journeyed through
the enormity these scars hold
it is divine beauty
true antlers of my heart
full heart
flat chest

LIVING WILD AND FREE

beyond life and death
is freedom

full circle

so it has come full circle
the exhaustion
the mass
the testing
the diagnosis
the treatment
the surgeries
the death
the rebirth
all of it encompassed in
love
beauty
joy
fear
pain
demise
duality
the quest took magic
of the forest
of life
of love
of community
of healing
to bring my soul back
to its body
desire for life
feeling every moment
not avoiding
rather welcoming it all in
with grace
to return
home
within

yew tree magic

i wrapped my arms
around your beautiful bark
filled with vibrance
i thanked you for your natural remedies
and those who discovered
your healing properties
the forest called me to you
to heal in the intoxicating technicolor greens
amongst cool moist soils
where you stood strong and wild
i felt your power inside me
and again outside me
in nature
the yew tree bark was infused within my body
your magic hung in chemotherapy bags
as the medicine taxol
the magic of your bark evicted cancer cells
from their residence in my body
and also caused debilitating
bone crushing pain
i was meant to thank you
where you lived firmly planted
in the pacific northwest forestlands
emotions flooded my system as we met
both in the infusion chair
and again on washington island soils
tears of joy
streamed from my eyes
for all you have gifted me
thank you for coming full circle with me
from life
to death
to life again
rooted in love
graced with gratitude
for this life
from a mystical
mighty tree

becoming water

will you accept all cancer has taught you

all the lessons in detaching
opening space to receive
leaving control
for the gift of freedom

can you accept living in the unknown

surfing life's mysterious ways
letting her move you through life
finding stillness inside
instead of grasping for it elsewhere
this life is a precious gift
always changing
eventually
the feels of comfort
are no longer
and the uncomfortable
becomes all you need
the unattached
becomes your spark of aliveness

this is the mystery
this is the gift

be as the water teaches
fluid in motion
it breaks the grit
smooths rocks to silky sand
let waves of grace
assist in the ever changing
beauty
of becoming
the flow
of water

the world through new eyes

the lens has been cleared
details amplify
art radiates
the energetic field becomes more visible
with these new eyes
comes a world
never before seen
and one which many
will never see

all things feel different
and the mind traps itself
in constant comparisons
between the almost
should haves
could have beens
would haves
but with this changed perspective
comes an acceptance
of life's fluidity
it feels foreign and fresh
with a reminder of courage
one learns how to trust again
how to observe
the constantly changing
slowly releasing the almost
should haves
could haves
would haves
to embrace
the now haves

the journey is
to remain no victim
to the old lens
in this current view
of now

journey inward

the uncomfortable feeling
of one breath before a dive
the body stretching in places never before felt
and the beauty
of learning how to relax into the feeling
as it takes you for a ride
to new places within being
deeply
rooted
anchored down strong
to reach freedom upward
growing inward
to ripple outward
journeying through
the captivating darkness
full of amazement and wonder
cracking open of self
to the mystery
where abundance reins
and the unknown
becomes a radical gift
for a bleeding soul
beyond the ego
there are no i's
in fully living
welcome to
deep lvng
life
beyond
the ego

finally free

relief does arrive
following a long arduous journey
it tastes of a flower's nectar
of a boundless expansion of abundance
the body's cells no longer buzz with fear
but rather are bathed in peace
breath is felt deep within the body again
without pain
whispers of the divine become audible
no longer silenced by a spiraling anxious mind
worries of reoccurrence loop
but each continually shortens in existence
joy blossoms in detailed moments
time becomes the ultimate gift
that responds to your creation
trepidation no longer grips your being
darkness sheds
light radiates
living is no longer affliction
worry wilts
clarity returns
how beautiful it is
to feel rebirth
to appreciate life
to be here now
in this magical experience
beyond life and death
is freedom
to
be
love

gratitude

It is with a heart full of gratitude that I acknowledge those who have helped to support this creation of artwork and channeled musings.

The tribal community- I am grateful for the collection of beings that surround me in love through so many ways during this cancer journey and beyond. I love y'all tremendously.

Family- I'm so grateful for all your unwavering support. Your love has been an anchor for my soul. Thank you for seeing me, always. I love you.

Shane Lasby- your love in supporting my journey has been such a gift to receive. Thank you for being a mirror of love's greatest depths.

The Powell family- thank you for providing a sacred space for me to channel this book (James, Raegan, Macy and Hayden). Within these pages are Washington forest soils.

Amanda McLenon- thank you for editing this collection of musings and for teaching me about the many riches of true friendship.

Book tribe- thank you to all who helped in proof reading, editing, formatting, as well as sharing testimonials (Joseph Tomarchio, Sundi Herring, Amanda McLenon, Loren Dupuis, Lee Beasley, Andrea Boyd and Shane Lasby).

Life in the mystery- I am grateful for spirit, for love, for this life. Thank you thank you thank you. I bow in gratitude to all that is, that was, and that is to come.

To you- thank you for connecting, sharing, loving, and being.

about the author

Melannie holds experience as a dive instructor, published marine scientist, and yoga teacher. She is passionate about inspiring connections with each other, within ourselves, and with our planet. She earned a Masters of Science degree in Marine Science from Hawaii Pacific University as well as a Bachelor of Science in Zoology from Michigan State University. As a triple negative breast cancer survivor diagnosed at age 35, she carries the BRCA1 gene mutation. The timeless art of writing has been an integral part of everything she does; like the water that flows through all she is fortunate to create. She shares her experiences through the potent energy of print with the intention of inspiring connection by feeling deeply within the golden thread of community.

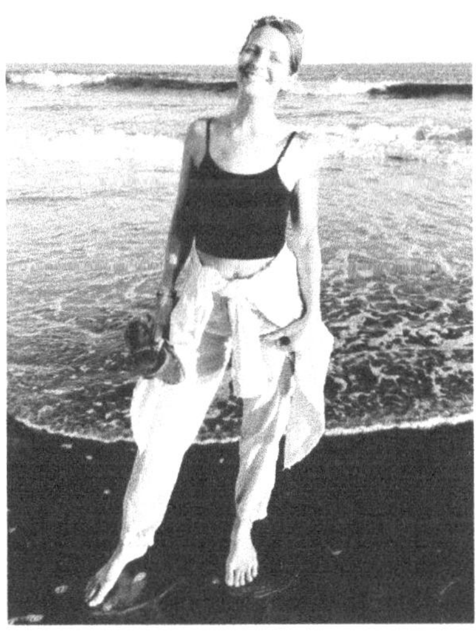

For more information, explore her website:
www.melanniebachman.com

www.ingramcontent.com/pod-product-compliance
Lightning Source LLC
Chambersburg PA
CBHW012041140726
47991CB00011B/3231